Hair Care Guide

Beginner's Guide to Hair Care for All Hair Types and Colors for Men and Women So You Can Have Gorgeous and Healthy Hair Year-Round

By Joan Dermody

© **Copyright 2020 - All rights reserved.**

The content contained within this book may not be reproduced, duplicated or transmitted without direct written permission from the author or the publisher.

Under no circumstances will any blame or legal responsibility be held against the publisher or author for any damages, reparation, or monetary loss due to the information contained within this book. Either directly or indirectly.

Legal Notice:

This book is copyright protected. This book is only for personal use. You cannot amend, distribute, sell, use, quote or paraphrase any part, or the content within this book, without the consent of the author or publisher.

Disclaimer Notice:

Please note the information contained within this document is for educational and entertainment purposes only. All effort has been executed to present accurate, up to date and reliable, complete information. No warranties of any kind are declared or implied. Readers acknowledge that the author is not engaging in the rendering of legal, financial, medical or professional advice. The content within this book has been derived from various sources. Please consult a licensed professional before attempting any techniques outlined in this book.

By reading this document, the reader agrees that under no

circumstances is the author responsible for any losses, direct or indirect, which are incurred as a result of the use of information contained within this document, including, but not limited to, —errors, omissions, or inaccuracies.

Contents

Chapter 1: 5 Ways to Minimize Dandruff 1
    Use shampoo 1
    Aloe Vera 2
    Apple Cider Vinegar 2
    Coconut Oil 3
    Go Organic 3

Chapter 2: Curly Hair Care Tips 5
    Love It 5
    Look after It 6
    Work It 7

Chapter 3: Easy Steps to Taking Care Of Your Hair 8
    Go Natural 8
    Condition 9
    Allow it to Shine 9

Chapter 4: Hair Care Tips for Guys 11
    Hair Shampoo and Conditioner 11
    Homemade Remedies 12
    Styling 13

Chapter 5: Hair Care Tips for Red Heads 14
    Select the Right Color 14
    Hair Shampoo and Conditioner 15
    Henna 15

Chapter 6: Tips for Great Blonde Hair Care 17
    Get The Yellow Out 17
    Condition 18

- Know When It's Not For You 19

Chapter 7: Things You Have to Learn About Loss Of Hair 20
- What It Is 20
- Conditions 21
- Choices 22

Chapter 8: Stunning Hair From The Inside Out 23
- Vitamins 23
- Food and Snacks 24

Chapter 9: Hair Care Per Person 26
- Straight vs Curly 26
- Blonde vs. Dark, With A Little Bit of Red 27
- Organic vs Non-organic 27

Chapter 10: Tips for Shiny Hair 29
- Protect 29
- Wash 30
- Condition 30
- Attempt Less Coloring 30
- Shiny You. 31

Chapter 11: Hair Care for Individuals With Serious Allergic Reactions ... 32
- Read All Labels, Whenever 32
- Warn Your Stylist 33
- Homemade Hair Care 34

Chapter 12: The Very Best Hair Care Beauty Parlor Treatments 35
- Scalp Massage 35
- Hair Mask 36
- Deep Conditioner 36
- Oil Treatment 37
- Facial With Scalp Massage 37

Chapter 13: 5 Tips for Supermodel Hair 39
    Condition 39
    Blow Dry 40
    Design 40
    Tease 41
    Attemp Something New 41

Chapter 14: Brunette and Black Hair Care Tips 42
    Color and Makeup 42
    Shine On 43
    Brunette Tips 44

Chapter 15: Romantic Hair Care Ideas 45
    Provide A Hair Care Present 45
    Offer Each Other Scalp Massages 46

Chapter 16: Summertime Hair Care 48
    Protect 48
    Brighten up 49
    Block the Sun 49
    Water 50
    Treatments 50

Thank you for buying this book and I hope that you will find it useful. If you will want to share your thoughts on this book, you can do so by leaving a review on the Amazon page, it helps me out a lot.

Chapter 1: 5 Ways to Minimize Dandruff

Dandruff is identified by the flakiness and scratchiness of the scalp. You can constantly talk to your dermatologist to determine the issue and for solutions that assist treat it. You might not even have dandruff; your present hair item, consisting of conditioner and shampoo, might be aggravating your scalp. So, attempt changing your item initially to non-dandruff hair shampoo and conditioner. See if the flakiness disappears. Stress could be a primary cause behind dandruff, so make certain that you attempt unwinding strategies daily to minimize your levels of stress.

Use shampoo

Wash your hair with warm to cool water. Attempt to use a moderate hair shampoo for a couple of weeks, and in case you do not see any outcomes, utilize an anti-dandruff hair shampoo. You ought to see an enhancement in 4-6 weeks. Don't use alcohol-based items, or any other styling items up until the dandruff subsides. Rather, utilize a leave-in conditioner.

Aloe Vera

You have to alleviate your scalp since it is inflamed and red, so attempt Aloe Vera. Rub the gel onto the scalp and maintain it there overnight. Make sure to change your pillowcase.

Apple Cider Vinegar

Attempt putting 2 tablespoons of Apple Cider Vinegar onto your scalp, or lemon juice, or perhaps attempt a mix of both. Leave it on for as long as you want, approximately 20 minutes to an hour ought to work, and after that, shampoo.

Coconut Oil

Coconut Oil is a calming and moderate option in alleviating dandruff. You can work it through your hair. After a couple of days, the dandruff ought to be gone.

Go Organic

You can utilize different herbs consisting of rosemary, ginger or thyme. You can blend rosemary and ginger with olive oil, individually and rub it onto the scalp. Tea could be made and after that, rubbed onto the scalp and shampooed. The Thyme oil is antibacterial and could be boiled and left on your hair.

You can likewise attempt to get rid of dandruff from the inside out. Cut down on unhealthy food, or remove it entirely from your eating plan. Attempt consuming yogurt. Likewise, incorporate more vegetables and fruits and milk. If the dandruff issue continues, or any of these solutions make the issue even worse, stop and look for medical attention. You wish to make certain it is, as a matter of fact, dandruff you handling. If it is another skin problem, it is going to be dealt with utilizing various solutions.

Chapter 2: Curly Hair Care Tips

Primary guideline for curly hair: enjoy it! It constantly astounds me when individuals with naturally curly hair do not entirely enjoy it. A lot of ladies go to extreme measures to get straight hair when they have something so terrific currently. Continuously aligning your hair with a flat iron can trigger considerable heat damage, and please do not get long-term hair straightening treatments performed.

Love It

Your naturally curly hair is lovely. Whether it is short, long, tight curls, or loose waves, you have numerous straight-haired ladies wanting they had simply a little bit of what you have! Long curly hair, specifically when healthy, could be very appealing. Guy frequently link sexiness with hair and see big hair to be really attractive. If a girl has actually wild yet managed curls, lots of guys are drawn to that appearance.

Look after It

The most essential thing for curly hair is conditioning. Frizzy, unmanageable natural curls can quickly be subdued by utilizing a conditioner created particularly for curly hair. Likewise, deep condition your curls one time a week, with homemade conditioners or beauty salon purchased treatments. Likewise, utilize a shine serum blended with a leave-in conditioner for a terrific curl appearance. Stiff curls that do not move aren't as fantastic as a curl which you are able to run your fingers through as it remains shaped. You can likewise blend leave-in with your mousse or gel to protect against the undesirable sticky appearance. Dry your hair upside down, on low and constantly utilize a diffuser. It is much better to allow your curls to dry naturally, however.

Work It

Now that you have actually got the curls you have actually constantly desired, flaunt them. When your hair is entirely dry, carry a little shine spray and gently mist the ended product. Whether you have long or short curls, if you like them, other individuals are going to like them and see them. It is necessary to be self-assured in yourself. Other individuals acknowledge and react to this quality. So, if you like your curls and stop speaking about just how much you wish to alter them and rather accept them, other individuals are going to like them too. You may even have a couple of the straight-haired gals wanting much more that they were ordained to have your curls, even if just for a day!

Chapter 3: Easy Steps to Taking Care Of Your Hair

Wish to know a few of the simplest actions for taking care of your hair? Attempt letting go of a couple of your hair items, or regimens and offer your hair a break!

Go Natural

Among the very best things you may do to look after your hair is to allow your hair to breathe, simply a bit. Attempt it for a week, and even simply a day and notice if you like the outcome. You pull, and blow-dry and heat your hair daily, picture what those little strands of hair have to handle. Still, you do not want to let it all go. You, in fact, may wish to emphasize your features by devoting additional time to a new style of makeup. Keep on washing your hair, and if you find the time, include a leave-in conditioner and allow it to air dry. You will find that this works particularly well for curly hair. In case your hair is wavy, you can use a wide-tooth comb to form it into a loose bun. In case you are dealing with a straight hair, you can pull it back into a chic ponytail.

Condition

Conditioning is crucial when it comes to hair care. Utilize an ordinary lightweight moisturizing conditioner regularly, along with utilizing a heavy deep conditioner for 15 minutes per week. The conditioner you use will depend upon your hair type and your particular preference. If you don't like the feeling of having too much hair product on your hair, then go with a lighter conditioner. If your hair is thick, then utilize a thick conditioner.

Allow it to Shine

Even when you allow your hair to naturally dry in order to enhance your hair care routine, it is still possible for your hair to shine. You can effortlessly achieve the shine by administering a shine hair serum to your hair. Make certain that you utilize this sparingly, less than a dime, or your hair is going to look greasy. Once the air drying is done, use a shine spray to achieve a polished appearance.

Chapter 4: Hair Care Tips for Guys

Okay men, be truthful, just how much do you truly appreciate your hair? Do you devote more time to your hair than your sweetheart does? Are your friends likewise offering you a difficult time since you have to have your hair on point for the big game? Or do you simply enjoy having your hair to look great? If you responded to any of these inquiries, then carry on with this part.

Hair Shampoo and Conditioner

A great hair shampoo has 4 standard qualities, it cleans the hair of debris and oil, it works in soft and hard water, it does not aggravate the skin, and it maintains the scalp and hair in natural excellent- looking condition. You may not wish to utilize a conditioner, since you're a man, however, you ought to! Numerous conditioners consist of lanolin, proteins, veggie oil, and herbs, and they are created to bring back natural oils and hydrate the hair. Leave in-condition are a terrific option too, and still offers some style.

Homemade Remedies

Eggs supply your body with protein, and they can likewise function as a hair shampoo. I do not suggest doing this every day, possibly one time a week or month. You just beat the egg in a bowl, and administer to the hair in a lather. Then clean your hair in cold or warm water. Do not utilize warm water, unless you desire scrambled eggs on your scalp! Utilize a lemon rinse, squeeze approximately half of the lemon within a cup. Olive oil is likewise a terrific treatment. Administer an ounce of olive oil to shampooed hair and place a steaming warm towel on your head. Leave it for approximately 15 minutes and wash.

Styling

I constantly think that less is more when it concerns guys's hair styling. The end outcome, when you have actually wrapped up styling, ought to never ever look done to death, or too styled. Guy's hair looks much better if you appear like you showered, utilized a smidgen of product, and start the day. This depends upon the texture and length of your hair. In case you have curly hair you might wish to utilize a mousse. For straight hair, attempt gel. Pomades work effectively to maintain your hair in place, however, it could be extremely sticky. Hair creams likewise work well and are an excellent option to utilize if you wish to run your fingers through your hair, or if you desire another person to!

Chapter 5: Hair Care Tips for Red Heads

Red could be among a few of the most lovely and clearly special colors you can get. A few of the most gorgeous mythical characters had red hair; even reading about the hair color is vibrant in one's head. Whether you are a natural redhead, or not, terrific hair care is important for this specific color. You desire your hair to be glossy and instead of a dull color, you desire it to flitter like a flame or the glossy red apple that lured Adam. Perhaps Eve was a redhead.

Select the Right Color

In case you are a natural red head, then you most likely have a paler complexion. Ensure that you emphasize your skin, and use make up to properly show your hair color. Attempt various brand names and items to see which works finest for you. Red hair is powerful, so rather, utilize slight dewy makeup colors which make your skin gleam. Just For Redheads provides a range of makeup colors created for redheads.

Hair Shampoo and Conditioner

Constantly utilize a hair shampoo that is developed for red hair. You can likewise discover conditioners that are particularly for red hair. Look for one that is hydrating and does not weigh down the hair, as red hair tends to be frizzier than other colors.

Henna

Red hair color is the sole real color that arises from Henna. There are numerous henna items that are offered. Constantly go over the item description and make certain it consists of nourishing and natural components. Abundant red hair could be among the most noticeably gorgeous colors. It is incredible, due to the fact that it is not seen extremely frequently. Among the most comprehensive methods to highlight your hair is to likewise wear the appropriate colors that just accentuate your natural appeal. So if you discover natural henna items that can highlight the inner shine, you are going to definitely draw in a great deal of favorable attention. Perhaps you'll even lure a few of those lookers.

Chapter 6: Tips for Great Blonde Hair Care

The very best pointer for blonde hair care is to obtain the appropriate color! Blonde is the trickiest of all of them. There is undoubtedly the unreasonable preconception that goes along with being a blonde. Apart from the psychological flack that lots of blondes get, in case you have the incorrect blonde shade, it is not going to do anything for you.

Get The Yellow Out

The outright worse issue for blondes is obtaining a rich blonde color and maintaining the yellow out. Regardless of what, yellow is created for school buses, not your hair! It has actually never ever been a natural color, and it does not appear excellent. The very best method to obtain blonde hair, with either all-over color or highlights, is to discover a fantastic stylist. It is more difficult than you may believe. Somehow, one either understands blonde hair or they do not. Communicate with your beautician over precisely what it is you desire. Do not be shy. Introduce photos of what you do desire, and tell them no yellow! Numerous people state toner is going to take it out, however, often utilizing a toner can turn the hair more yellow. Utilizing a purple hair shampoo, is a terrific option.

Condition

When hair is handled with bleach, it could be incredibly destructive. You can utilize homemade conditioners with recipes that consist of mayonnaise, olive oil, eggs, or avocados; the choices are limitless. Regardless, however, utilize a conditioner daily. You can even utilize a leave-in for much better outcomes and deep condition one time a week at least.

Know When It's Not For You

Blonde is not for everybody. It is one color that either is for you or isn't. In case you have white-blonde hair naturally: fortunate you. You can pick in between dark and ash blonde to the gorgeous appearance of well-done platinum. Have the appropriate makeup for the blonde hair and tone it down a bit, the hair is typically strong enough. In case you have black hair naturally, blonde is more than likely not going to look great; rather, discover an excellent dark abundant color.

Chapter 7: Things You Have to Learn About Loss Of Hair

35 million guys deal with loss of hair every year in the US. 20 percent of guys in their twenties struggle with losing their hair and that increases to half of guys in their fifties. Both women and men deal with loss of hair and the most scientific explanation for why is genetic. 60 percent of ladies deal with some hair loss by menopause.

What It Is

Anagen is the growth stage. Hair is able to grow for as much as 6 years, based upon your age. Right after adolescence in the teen years, one experiences the largest amount of hair growth, due to a high rate of hormonal agents. Catagen is the stage through which the follicle closes down and Telogen is the resting stage. At the Telogen stage hair stops growing entirely. The hair follicle diminishes. If the hair follicle perishes, then there is female and male pattern baldness. The explanation that ladies lose their hair too, is due to the fact that females are born with androgens, the male hormonal agents that trigger loss of hair, if you acquire them genetically, along with estrogens that have the opposite impact. You might be shedding your hair in case you see a lot of hair on your pillow, or within the shower drain.

Conditions

Cicatricial alopecia is an irreparable type of loss of hair related to scarring on the scalp. Genetic alopecia is the lack of hair on the scalp and it can happen alone, or with another condition. Symptomatic alopecia is the hair loss because of signs of a psychogenic cause like basic health, skin or scalp infections, and tension. Other reasons why someone may deal with loss of hair is due to bad nutrition and depression.

Choices

There are numerous choices that a person can make the most of when it concerns loss of hair. Propecia and Rogaine are 2 of the very popular loss of hair medications. Cortisone can likewise promote hair growth. Hair transplantation is another choice. Hair weaving is likewise readily available, this is the treatment of weaving or sewing a base into the staying hair on the scalp, and after that, weaving human hair into the structure. Loss of hair could be a tough thing to handle, whether you are a female or male. You can additionally consult your physician about choices or issues concerning loss of hair.

Chapter 8: Stunning Hair From The Inside Out

Do you desire lovely hair? Is everything that you're attempting topically not helping you? Are you conditioning regularly and utilizing non-damaging hair items? Then let's attempt to draw out your natural appeal from within by providing you gorgeous hair from the inside out.

Vitamins

Vitamins are an excellent method to assist you to keep your hair, and protect against loss of hair, and likewise enhance the state of your hair today. Ginkgo Biloba, vitamin E and anti-oxidants are great supplements for your hair. Biotin, which could be consumed orally in tablet form or injected, is thought to reinforce nails, skin and hair. Omega-3 fats enhance blood circulation and nourish the root. Foods which contain a wealth of Omega-3 are tuna, salmon, mackerel, mahi-mahi, and swordfish. Canola oil, olive oil and nuts, featuring pecans and walnuts offer Omega-3 fats by means of land-based sources.

Food and Snacks

A few of the very best healthy treats and food for terrific hair consist of the following:

- Sardines and Salmon, Eggs

- Lentils/Wheat Bran and Germ

- Watercress and Spinach

- Seaweed, Rice.

- Cantaloupe, Citrus fruits, Blueberries

- Walnuts and Almonds, Sunflower Seeds

- Figs, Bananas, Apricots

- Raspberries, Oranges, Strawberries

- Prunes and Raisins

- Low-fat yogurt and skim milk

- Snack bars and whole grain cereal

Hair is comprised of protein, so an exceptional eating plan, loaded with sulfur abundant foods, like beans, dairy, milk, eggs and fish are terrific for your hair. To enhance your hair's shine, you can consume ginger, chickpeas, apples, olive oil, and ground flaxseed or oil. Broccoli, tomatoes, cabbage, carrots, and string beans are excellent veggies to consume to promote greater hair care. Green tea is abundant in anti-oxidants and works in dealing with male pattern baldness. Oatmeal is likewise suggested to utilize as a hair mask, it works due to the fact that it exfoliates skin cells, and the hydrolyzed oat protein functions as a volumizer for the hair shaft. A multivitamin is an exceptional choice to feature in your inner beauty hair care routines. Routine working out and having the ability to destress might likewise add to your inner hair care journey. You may simply discover when you are unwinded and taking great care of yourself both mentally and physically, your hair is going to go to fantastic lengths.

Chapter 9: Hair Care Per Person

Hair care is individual. Hair care is likewise distinct for everybody. This is due to the fact that everybody's hair is distinct. You can have 2 sisters from the identical parents having totally distinct texture, color and design of hair. For that reason, hair care needs to be customized for every individual.

Straight vs Curly

2 really various kinds of hair are straight and curly. One is able to dry in a natural way and have no body, while the other is going to have plenty of body while being rowdy. Conditioner and shampoo are both crucial in both of these hair types. You might wish to stay with a lighter conditioner in case you come with straight fine hair and choose a heavy dense conditioner for extremely curly hair.

Blonde vs. Dark, With A Little Bit of Red

This truly is everything about color. The appropriate color on the appropriate individual can make all the distinction. The terrific thing is that you do not need to be a natural-born. Pick the color that is really the appropriate one for your complexion. Color likewise shows in the makeup you use, and the clothing you don. For red heads this is definitely vital. Purples and greens generally look great on pale-skinned red heads.

Organic vs Non-organic

Within current years, the spread of natural hair care lines has actually definitely proliferated. Non- natural mainstream lines have actually likewise kept on growing. You can discover and get lines of products that are devoted to environment-friendly practices and have terrible items; and you can discover mainstream lines that do not include environmentally friendly practices and have terrific items and vice versa. You need to do your homework on both kinds of lines. With the web you can check out reviews and choose which item work ideally for you. You can likewise discover more about the business and the kinds of components they utilize. This is crucial, particularly if you dislike specific components.

Chapter 10: Tips for Shiny Hair

Have you constantly desired smooth, glossy hair? It matters not if you are a brunette, blonde, or redhead. It likewise does not matter if you are a guy, girl, or teen. You can have glossy hair, and you can have it low-cost. There are simply a couple of basic pointers you require to obtain that soft shine hair, and it's through remarkable hair care.

Protect

The very best method to enhance the shininess of your hair does not suggest to do less, it simply suggests to protect it. Consider all of the tension your hair goes through daily. Hair gets drawn back, brushed, heated, moved, and even ripped out. So attempt just utilizing heating items, consisting of a curing iron or flat iron every other day.

Wash

Shampoo your hair. Some individuals state not to clean every day, others state that it is alright. Do what you feel comfy with, however, keep it tidy. Rinses with cold water stop your hair from getting damaged by really warm water.

Condition

Whether it is a homemade conditioner, or a costly beauty parlor item, condition your hair. Condition regularly and at least one time a week. Olive oil warmed up with your preferred essential oil is a fast and terrific choice. The Olive Oil hydrates and offers a terrific fragrance.

Attempt Less Coloring

Put your beauty parlor visits further apart. It may appear radical when we like our hair newly highlighted, however, it may be much better for your hair to spread them out. If you like your routine beauty parlor visits, in between coloring or highlighting sessions, book a deep conditioning procedure. Likewise, utilize color-enhancing conditioners and shampoos to extend the effect those highlights can provide.

Shiny You.

Search for conditioner, shampoo and items which have tea tree or other essential oils. One hundred percent olive oil and jojoba oil are likewise terrific options that could be used. You can likewise utilize serum and shine spray. Ensure you do not put these items on your root, as they can make your hair appear oily. Do it yourself or ask your partner or spouse to perform a scalp massage, it is going to promote natural oils, and is likewise really peaceful. It is likewise thought that rubbing your scalp can promote hair development!

Chapter 11: Hair Care for Individuals With Serious Allergic Reactions

Are you badly allergic to specific items or foods? In case you are, then you have to be additionally cautious when it pertains to looking for hair care items.

Read All Labels, Whenever

Checking out labels is among the most effective methods to avoid an allergy. If you understand the items that you dislike, you need to be specifically cautious of skin and hair care lines, due to the fact that much of them consist of food components, like nuts and berries. Nut allergic reactions are among the most fatal allergies to have. Anybody who has nut allergy understand that they have to search for macadamia nut oil, sweet almond oil and even kukui nut oil. It ends up being harder if you aren't sure if the item is a nut you are really allergic to. The most ideal thing to do is to be on the side of caution and do not utilize that item.

Warn Your Stylist

You have to alert your stylist, just as you would a waiter about your allergic reaction. They may forget and get an item that may be fantastic for your hair, which might be possibly hazardous for you. Make certain you are sharp and make certain the stylist does not utilize any brand-new item you are uncertain of. Topical allergic reactions could be as extreme as ingested allergic reactions. Touching a raw egg for somebody who is allergic can trigger his/her hand to puff up. Touching a nut, and after that, touching your eye can trigger a response of your eye swelling shut. Even breathing in can trigger a response from extreme to acute. So having a stylist place hair shampoo on your hair and you even breathing in the fumes from the irritant can trigger you to have asthma or another response.

Homemade Hair Care

Among the important things about homemade hair care that somebody with allergic reactions has to comprehend is that lots of are made exclusively with nuts, eggs and even dairy. Straight eggs and mayo could be utilized as an excellent replacement to condition and tidy hair. Numerous homemade creams consist of milk, yogurt and sweet almond oil. You can utilize replacements and you need to. Never ever risk an allergic reaction, especially if it might trigger you to enter into anaphylactic shock.

Chapter 12: The Very Best Hair Care Beauty Parlor Treatments

Typically, when individuals consider the beauty parlor, images aside from leisure pop into their mind. They just see hair dropping to the ground, bleach combusting the hair, heat coming off of the head, hair being converted into all various abnormal tones. That does not need to be the case, however. Lots of beauty parlors have not just styling services, however, likewise great deep conditioning treatments to enhance the total appearance of your hair.

Scalp Massage

I can not imagine anything more peaceful than having my head massaged. I might lay back and have my head rubbed for hours. Including in a hair shampoo, conditioner and blow-dry is a great touch; however, it is the scalp massage I like. A stylist either delights in doing this or does not and it can be seen easily. Ensure your stylist understands if they are using adequate pressure or excessive, and ask them to change.

Hair Mask

The hair mask components are going to differ based upon a particular beauty parlor. If a beauty parlor brings their own line of product, they are going to include that into your hair mask. Protein-rich seaweeds, and sea kelp are typically integrated into the hair mask and are developed to deal with color-treated and dry hair. Numerous likewise include numerous vitamins. Rather than sitting beneath the clothes dryer, if the weather condition allows it, ask if you can sit in the sun.

Deep Conditioner

This is a typical treatment used at beauty parlors. A heavy or thick deep-penetrating conditioner is put on your head, often in addition to a relaxing scalp massage. You can typically select to choose in between a deep protein treatment and a deep moisturizing treatment.

Oil Treatment

An oil treatment could be put on your scalp to lower dandruff or condition and hydrate your hair. The oils could be selected by you, and you ought to specify your choices if you have any. The stylist must allow you to sniff the essential oil before it is put on your scalp.

Facial With Scalp Massage

Some estheticians provide a scalp massage to go along with your facial. Ensure the esthetician utilizes an item you are not sensitive to, as numerous facials can trigger breakouts. After the esthetician exfoliates, cleans, hydrates and massages your face, and generally arms, you may be offered a scalp massage. No matter what you do: say yes!

Chapter 13: 5 Tips for Supermodel Hair

Supermodels appear to have the most lovely hair, don't they? Well, you might have the ability to get that identical look via these supermodel techniques and fantastic hair care. Keep in mind that lots of models have extensions, and that is what develops much of their body and volume. In case you do not possess dense hair, or extensions, you might not have the identical result, however, there is no issue with giving it a shot.

Condition

Whenever you understand you will be utilizing a great deal of heat, or including tension to your hair, ensure it is conditioned, both prior and after. Utilize a thicker conditioner and deep condition after you have actually attempted the new appearance. Likewise, seal your hair with a heat protector. Many lines bring them. If you can't discover one, utilize a leave-in conditioner.

Blow Dry

Blow-dry your hair with your head turned over on high, you can include a little bit of hair spray to include volume, not excessively, though. Include a volume-enhancing mousse to promote that large hair appearance. Blow-dry in areas to ensure you get out any undesirable kinks.

Design

As soon as your hair is dry, brush through it carefully and put your hair half up utilizing a clip. Spray the hair which is loose and safely put rollers into your hair. Perform this layer by layer, till all of your hair is rolled. After that, with low volume, blow-dry every roller. Maintain the rollers in for approximately 15 minutes. Take out the rollers without brushing them. Spray on a gentle hair spray for additional hold after you rub your fingers carefully through your hair. Don't brush.

Tease

you ought to constantly leave them desiring more, so go on, be a tease. In case you get a bit bored with supermodel hair, switch it up a little. You may put it half up and tease the top for additional volume utilizing a fine tooth-teasing comb.

Attemp Something New

Simply attempt something brand-new. In case you are daring and in your twenties, go for the low pigtails attractive appearance. They may be extremely attractive. In case you are older, it is going to work too. Bind with a rubber band that is the identical color as your hair, and maintain them low, beneath your ears, near your neck.

Chapter 14: Brunette and Black Hair Care Tips

Dark hair is mystical. That is the initial thing I consider when I see dark hair. Often brunettes think they take the clever rear seats to the hot blonde buddy or the wild red head. That's a thing to be happy with! Dark hair may be a gorgeous mix, especially when the appropriate shade has actually been discovered.

Color and Makeup

Brunette is likewise the hair color that can have such a broad range of choices when it concerns clothes and makeup, depending upon the complexion of the brunette. Light honey highlights may be included to chestnut brown hair for that additional stir. Often brunette hair appears much better without highlights, particularly darker brunettes. Brunettes can likewise be on 2 really reverse sides of the spectrum. One can have dark brown to black hair and a velvety white skin tone that is emphasized magnificently with a red lip. The caramel color brunette with normally blonde skin can don remarkable smoky eye makeup, with a naked lip, and appear bronzed, without anybody analyzing tanning methods.

Shine On

Black hair is probably the shiniest. Numerous Asian ladies are recognized for extremely glossy thick hair. Eating plan might have a great deal to do with the health and shine of a brunette's hair, however, some items can definitely assist! For African-American ladies who deal with coarse hair, olive oil conditioners could be a terrific option; and that natural tight curl can likewise be extremely stunning. There are numerous brunette conditioners, hair shampoos and items that may make your brown hair shine.

Brunette Tips

Some pointers to remember when dying your hair brown, is that the abundant shade might fade. Pick color improving conditioners and weekly treatments that lengthen that lovely brown shine. You can constantly darken or lighten a brunette color, if thinking about going black, attempt a medium to dark brown and proceed from there. Oftentimes the outcomes still preserve that feel of mystery.

Chapter 15: Romantic Hair Care Ideas

So, you never ever believed hair care might be so attractive, huh? Well, it could be if done correctly. If you are searching for excellent romantic ideas that you and your spouse, partner, boyfriend, girlfriend may do, hair care is among them. The result is helpful to both of you. You have a good time with the individual you appreciate, you can end up being more intimate, and your hair is going to look terrific.

Provide A Hair Care Present

For men, this is an excellent method to tell your woman you adore her. Do it the proper way, however. If your partner is constantly informing you she wishes to get her hair colored or highlighted, however, it's simply too costly, surprise her on Christmas, her birthday or another event and offer her this elegant present. If she currently has a set hairstylist that you understand she believes does an excellent job, purchase a present certificate at that beauty parlor with that individual. If you aren't certain, ask her buddies, or somebody she might have spoken to about this. And when you give it to her, utilize common sense, do not make it look like she has to get her hair done; inform her how you recall her stating she wished to get it done, so you did it for her. She is going to like it.

Offer Each Other Scalp Massages

You do not need to do it on the identical night; you can change it up, so the individual who is getting it can genuinely unwind. It's advised that the man does it initially, so the female understands this is genuine, and something she will need to follow through on, since you currently did. Ask her what her preferred fragrance is. If you actually wish to amaze her, you can blend jojoba or olive oil with rose, lavender or lemon to unwind. You might desire her to utilize sandalwood for you; it's a manly fragrance. Then set the mood by utilizing odorless or candle lights and light beeswax.

Then offer her the very best scalp massage you can think of. Be careful and rub her head in circular motions. Simply utilize your hands how you would touch the remainder of her body, and have fun with her hair. It is among the most intimate and peaceful times you may share.

Chapter 16: Summertime Hair Care

Hair ought to be changed through the summertime in the way you look after it. Hair care is incredibly vital throughout the summer season. Hair can end up being very dry and places like chlorinated swimming pools can induce damage to your hair.

Protect

If you are entering into a swimming pool or an ocean, you have to protect your hair from the destructive impacts of chlorine. You ought to constantly gently damp your hair prior to entering into the water. You can even lightly damp it with salt water or place a conditioner in your hair prior to swimming.

Brighten up

If you have blonde hair, among the important things you eagerly anticipate is the summertime, to organically lighten your hair. Just put lemon and olive oil onto your hair and sit outdoors. Do this regularly and you are going to observe that your hair is shinier and more workable. Many individuals do not enjoy the thought of administering lemon juice to hair as it could be drying. You can utilize the lemon juice though and blend it with sun block for your hair. Then you can offer yourself a weekly deep conditioning treatment, to bring the wetness back into your hair. You may have to deep condition two times a week to guarantee that adequate wetness is entering into your hair.

Block the Sun

Yes, utilize sunscreen on your hair. It is a fantastic method to prevent damage, along with stopping your scalp from burning. Lots of lines of the product provide a sun block to shield your hair.

Water

Consume water, it is an excellent method to guarantee you are hydrated and an excellent method to make your skin and hair radiate.

Treatments

Utilize a homemade rinse. When utilizing vinegar, mix it with herbs like lavender, lemon balm, chamomile, lemon verbena, or rose water to get rid of or tone down the vinegar odor. Mix one cup of apple cider vinegar with one cup of water, and a handful of mint leaves. Bring all of the components to a boil, strain and place into a container. Then merely massage onto your scalp, and all over your hair and keep it in.

I hope that you enjoyed reading through this book and that you have found it useful. If you want to share your thoughts on this book, you can do so by leaving a review on the Amazon page. Have a great rest of the day.

Printed in Poland
by Amazon Fulfillment
Poland Sp. z o.o., Wrocław